Sleep Apnoea

What is it? How to beat it, have a Better Rest, Fall Asleep Faster and Live a Transformed Life

© Copyright 2018 - All rights reserved.

The contents of this book may not be reproduced, duplicated or transmitted without direct written permission from the author. Under no circumstances will any legal responsibility or blame be held against the publisher for any reparation, damages, or monetary loss due to the information herein, either directly or indirectly.

Legal Notice:

This book is copyright protected. This is only for personal use. You cannot amend, distribute, sell, use, quote or paraphrase any part or the content within this book without the consent of the author.

Disclaimer Notice:

Please note the information contained within this document is for educational and entertainment purposes only. Every attempt has been made to provide accurate, up to date and reliable complete information. No warranties of any kind are expressed or implied. Readers acknowledge that the author is not engaging in the rendering of legal, financial, medical or professional advice. The content of this book has been derived from various sources. Please consult a licensed professional before attempting any techniques outlined in this book.

By reading this document, the reader agrees that under no circumstances are is the author responsible for any losses, direct or indirect, which are incurred as a result of the use of information contained within this document, including, but not limited to, —errors, omissions, or inaccuracies.

Table of Contents

Preface

So, we were all having a laugh at each other. Making fun of how one another slept. Some snored loud, some spoke in their sleep, some twitched like a rabbit, and now it was my daughter's turn to impersonate me.

"This is an impression of Daddy" she said,

"Snore Snore
Snore……………………………………………………………………
…….(silence)", and then she gasped as though she was taking in air for the first time after being drowned! And then they all laughed at me and I joined in, half worried.

"Do I really do that?" I said. They all nodded their head. Though I smiled I knew it was time that I did something about it.

I spoke to my wife that night and she collaborated the story. "You do it John, you give me heart attacks almost every night because I think you're not going to take another breath".

After a short time of research and a visit to the doctor within a couple weeks I was diagnosed with Sleep Apnoea. And thus began my search for a solution that would help me and all those who followed.

In this book I'll show you what I did to beat this condition and thus transform my life. And I want you to be able to do the same.

Prepare to be enlightened!

Let's get started.

Introduction

One day a work colleague asked me: "When was the last time you had a good night of sleep?". Though I felt tired and had been working through some tough deadlines in the city, I never thought it would be so obvious that I had problems sleeping. Maybe the blackish eye bags gave me in or my lack of attention during long meetings. Anyway, I knew I had to do something or else.

I hadn't told anyone apart from my wife, but I was waking with headaches almost every morning. I would open my eyes in the morning, try to keep as still as possible, and then ask myself the question "Is my head hurting this morning". Sometimes, as I would move my head it would be free of pain and I would have a good day. Most other days there was a slight niggle and I knew in my heart of hearts that the day would be a struggle. "Heavy Head", "Heavy Face", whatever you want to call it, it made me miserable.

For years I had been blaming it on my sinuses. The doctor had told me that I had chronic rhinitis that would flare up as and when, and that would lead to headaches. All I knew was that I was in pain, miserable, always tired and now people were beginning to see the results of my struggle at work.

I was never the kind of person that once I'd hit a pillow I would quickly fall asleep. But, due to all sorts of life events, my sleeping hours become shorter and shorter. And even when I would sleep 8 to 10 hours during long weekends, I would still find myself more tired than usual. There was something wrong and it had started to affect my personal and professional life. I would get angry very easily, lack focus and stamina, and everyone around me started to notice.

After the conversation with my colleague, it took me a few weeks to have another good night of sleep. I tried all sorts of conventional medicines and even some not so conventional medicines and therapies. Some had nasty effects on my body, while others would not last long and I had to keep on coming back for more. I increased my intake of caffeine in the office, but this just increased my outtake of explosive comments and breakdowns in my home.

So, it was that short family moment that made all the difference. The moment where we joked…about me dying 10 times in the middle of the night!

It worried me, and it drove me to do something about it. I realized in that one moment that I had one life to live. One season where my kids were the age they were, and that there was and a responsibility on me to do everything I could to not let this condition beat me.

To my surprise, after speaking to professionals, conducting comprehensive research, it was the simplest of changes in my lifestyle, and in my home, that had a long-lasting effect in the way that I would fall asleep, stay asleep and have a better rest during the night. It really changed my life for the better.

The simple fact is, that after implementing everything that I will share with you in this short book, I feel more energized, happier, fitter, and stronger. I look forward to opening the door of my room at the end of the day and falling sleep. I also spring to my feet in the morning to get back to work with a smile on my face, knowing that I have no pain, but I am free to face the day 100% fit.

As stated, I took some time to do my own research and tried some tips and tricks from friends and online sources. Found out that what worked for me didn't work for everyone else. I shared my secrets with family, friends and office-mates, but not all seemed convinced of my strategies to get a really effective restful sleep. So, I decided to gather everything I found that is helpful for others and me and put it all down in a notepad and share it. I am sure that these tips will be helpful for you as they were for me.

Try a little bit of everything and find what works the best for you. Here are a few tips on how I beat Sleep

Apnoea, and some general guidelines on how to rest better, fall asleep faster and live a transformed life. Once you have done reading through these, you will feel like you don't need to know anything else; everything you need to know is in here!

What is this... Sleep Apnoea?

The proper, full name for Sleep Apnoea is Obstructive Sleep Apnoea (OSA). You will be relieved to know that OSA is a relatively common condition and what basically happen is that the walls of the throat relax and narrow during sleep, interrupting normal breathing. This scared me, when I first found out but its ok, lets keep going.

It is the relaxing of these walls that lead to regularly interrupted sleep, which can have a major effect on your quality of life and increases the risk of developing certain other conditions.

If I am honest it was the risk of developing other conditions that drove me to research and caused me to make a change.

Physicians say that there are two types of Apnoea. **Apnoea** and **hypopnea.**

They are different because they take on different characteristics.

Apnoea

This is where the muscles and soft tissues in the throat relax and collapse sufficiently to cause a total blockage of the airway; it's called an apnoea when the airflow is blocked for 10 seconds or more. This is what I had!

The second type is called

Hypopnoea

This is a partial blockage of the airway that results in an airflow reduction of greater than 50% for 10 seconds or more.

It is said that people with OSA may experience repeated episodes of apnoea and hypopnoea throughout the night and that these events may occur around once every one or two minutes in severe cases.

The United Kingdom National Health Service state that "as many people with OSA experience episodes of both apnoea and hypopnoea, doctors sometimes refer to the condition as obstructive sleep apnoea-hypopnoea syndrome, or OSAHS."

The Giveaway signs of OSA

After research I found out that the common symptoms of OSA are often first highlighted by a partner, friend or family member who notices problems while you sleep. As mentioned, for me it was my wife….and then my kids…who subsequently took the micky!

Research also suggests that some of the common signs of OSA in someone sleeping can include:

- loud snoring
- noisy and labored breathing
- Some people with OSA may also experience night sweats and may wake up frequently during the night to urinate.
- Waking up with a very sore or dry throat.
- Occasionally waking up with a choking or gasping sensation.
- Sleepiness or lack of energy during the day.
- Sleepiness while driving.

- Forgetfulness, mood changes, and a decreased interest in sex
- Morning headaches.
- Restless sleep.

What basically happens is, during an episode, the lack of oxygen triggers your brain to pull you out of deep sleep – either to a lighter sleep or to wakefulness – so your airway reopens, and you can breathe normally.

It is because of these sleep interruptions you may feel very tired during the day. You'll usually have no memory of your interrupted breathing, so you may be unaware you have a problem. This was the case for me.

What Should I do About It?

When the condition was finally highlighted to me I went straight to my local GP. I would encourage you to do the same.

I will be honest with you, it was the long term affects that really drove me past the macho, "Ill deal with it myself" mentality.

Have a look for yourself. Some of the long-term effects are:

- Depression.
- High blood pressure.
- Stroke.
- Heart failure, irregular heart beats, and heart attacks.
- Diabetes.
- Worsening of ADHD.
- Headaches.

I told you it was serious! Get over yourself and get to the doctors!

Your doctor can check for other possible reasons for your symptoms and can arrange for an assessment of your sleep to be carried out through a local sleep center.

What Could be the Cause of this Condition?

There is the medical reason and then some practical reasons why Sleep Apnoea has appeared in your life.

The medical reason is that its normal for the muscles and soft tissues in the throat to relax and collapse to some degree while sleeping. For most people this doesn't cause breathing problems.

In people with Sleep Apnoea the airway has narrowed as the result of a number of factors, including:

- **Being Overweight** – extra body fat increases the bulk of soft tissue in the neck, which can place a strain on the throat muscles; excess stomach fat can also lead to breathing difficulties, which can make Sleep Apnoea worse. (We will talk about this one later)

- **Being 40 years of age or more**

- **Being of the Male Sex** – it's not known why OSA is more common in men than in women, but it may be related to different patterns of body fat distribution

- **Having a large neck** – men with a collar size greater than around 43cm (17 inches) have an increased risk of developing OSA

Additional Reasons Include:

- **Menopause (in women)** – the changes in hormone levels during the menopause may cause the throat muscles to relax more than usual
- **Alcohol** – drinking alcohol, particularly before going to sleep, can make snoring and sleep apnoea worse
- **Taking medicines with a sedative effect** – such as sleeping tablets or tranquillizers

- **Having an unusual inner neck structure** – such as a narrow airway, large tonsils, adenoids or tongue, or a small lower jaw

- **Nasal congestion** – OSA occurs more often in people with nasal congestion, such as a deviated septum, where the tissue in the nose that divides the two nostrils is bent to one side, or nasal polyps, which may be a result of the airways being narrowed

- **Smoking** – you're more likely to develop sleep apnoea if you smoke

- **Having OSA In the Family Tree** – there may be genes inherited from your parents that can make you more susceptible to OSA

So, What Now?

For me, as soon as I went to the Doctor, I knew what he was going to say. I'd done the research, I was just waiting for him to confirm what I already knew.

"You are carrying over 3 stone too much weight", he said.

I knew that already but hearing it from someone else wasn't a great experience. He might as well have said. "Move it fat man! don't come back here until you sort yourself out!"

It was this moment that got me moving, got me changing, got me researching and then implementing what I learnt, and this is what I am going to share with you.

After asking my wife whether she thought that I had Sleep Apnoea when we first married she had told me I did, so I knew that if I could some how loose this weight it would be a good start. From the next morning I was on it, I did everything I could to get the weight off and live heather. As well as implement what I am just about to share with you.

All I know is, Sleep Apnoea haunted me at night, and now I doesn't, thanks to my weight loss and also the steps that I will share with you now.

Read, digest and implement and I would love to hear your results.

It all starts the day before…

The Day Before

It all starts during the day and before you even get yourself into your favorite pajamas and ready to hit the valley of bed sheets. Imagine that you are a train, moving through your day at incredible speeds, trying to meet, and exceed expectations and schedules. Once you reach your final station, Dream Land, the faster you go, the harder it is to stop, right? Because your body may be tired and looking to rest, but your mind is still racing through what has happened to
you during the day and planning the day ahead.

I know that most of us really do lead high-octane lives with increasing stress levels and anxieties, many of which may be good in paving the way to success. Though at the end of the day, we are all the same and we all need to recycle those energies, allow our bodies to go through its own purification process and our own natural stages of sleep. A night of uninterrupted sleep allows your body to repair and rest its own muscles, to consolidate your memory and rest the brain. It will release hormones that regulate both your body's appetite and growth.

The first thing that you can do is to answer the following questions and keep these in your mind while you change your daily habits. Find whatever works best by increasing or reducing the amounts for each of these categories:

How many hours of sleep do you need? This is different for every person and at different times in our lives, but our bodies require more or less the same amount of hours, depending on our age. While children below 5 years old sleep most of the time, between 12 to 14 hours per day, children above 5 and up to 12 require around 10 hours of sleep. Teens, from 12 to 18 years old, still require long hours of good sleep to allow their bodies to grow and also to allow their increasing mental activity to find time to rest. They need as much as 10 hours of daily sleep. Adults can live healthy lives with 8 hours of sleep.

The older you get, the harder it is to actually sleep that many hours. This is mostly caused by the increasing demands of our lives and diverse responsibilities. If you can't sleep through the night, try to take daytime naps. Keep a diary of how many hours you sleep per day and how you feel when you wake up, during the day and before you sleep. This will allow you to gauge the amount of hours that you really need, without letting yourself sleep too much or too little.

What is your diet? If you eat too much or do not eat enough, your body will lack the nutrients and vitamins that it needs to fully function during the day. This means that at the end of the day it will feel restless and not comfortable. Foods that can help you to sleep better are: fish, due to being lighter than most meats and easier to digest; bananas are great because they have potassium and magnesium, which help to relax the muscles; chamomile is a great herb to drink as tea, its tranquilizing effects have been known for ages, you can trust your grandmother's advice on this; any food with high levels of calcium, like spinach, because it helps your body to create melatonin, a hormone that helps you to sleep. While on this note on calcium, milk is great for the same reasons, so no wonder why kids sleep better after a cup of warm milk.

What is your regular physical exercise? Exercise frequently, besides the fact that it will help you to have a healthier life. It will also help your body to reduce accumulated stress, recycle damaged cells that increase aging signs and all sorts of bodily waste. Exercise helps to control your body fat levels, build stronger bones as you sleep, relax your muscles, control blood pressure and increase your libido. All of which will help you to sleep better.

How much caffeine do you drink? You should also consider any energy inducing beverages, with alcohol or artificial stimulants, because these will affect your normal bodily rhythms. I still drink my coffee in the morning and I like to socialize around mojitos and daiquiris, but I know when to stop and what is already enough for me.

After checking all of these questions by keeping a daily journal of these activities, checking how they affect your sleep and how you feel rested during the day. Try to find your sweet spot; the right amount of each one that helps you get to sleep faster and sleep better.

Alongside this, try to avoid late night snacks. Do not eat anything that is to digest before you go to sleep. Otherwise, your body will be processing the food as you sleep. If you are hungry, drink some warm milk and cookies. Some psychologists have considered this may be directly connected to childhood memories and even with breastfeeding experiences.

Follow a strict schedule. Do not allow yourself to sleep at disorderly hours. Set yourself the discipline to sleep at a certain hour and wake up after a certain amount of hours. If you stay awake late into the night, your body will feel pressed to stay awake because naturally, after sundown, due to the lack of light, your body is already starting to get ready to sleep. Even if you don't have anything to do the next day, try to go to sleep at the same time every night. The same goes for waking up, even when you don't have anything to do. Do not stay in bed too long; it is as bad as sleeping too little.

As I said in the beginning, what may work for some does not work for others. Our bodies have different ways to handle our daily activities. We have different schedules and responsibilities. It took me some weeks to discipline myself into a sleeping schedule that actually works for me and is effective. I remember one day going to bed too early, ended up staying awake and bored in bed. I used to drink 5 to 6 cups of coffee daily. I tried to reduce it drastically in a week and ended up feeling more tired and stressed than usual. This process is a dialogue between you and your body; allow it to express to you and allow it to indulge sometimes in life's pleasures.

Don't worry or feel guilty for being happy and allowing yourself to eat, drink and sleep enough to give you the energy levels that you need to get you through the day. One last tip on this: let everyone around you know that you are trying new techniques and different lifestyle choices to improve your sleeping habits. They will surely understand if you are grumpy or tired some days, and they will surely provide the support you need to get through it.

In the Room, On the Bed

Unless you like to sleep on the sofa, the floor or you are camping, the magic happens in the room and on the bed. The ambiance in the room is very important as it can be conducive to help you fall asleep faster and have a restful night, or keep you awake. Think about how you feel when you enter a messy room, and how different it is when you enter a room that is neatly organized, smells good, is quite and well lit. The same principal can be applied to the bed. Some of the best nights of sleep I had were in hotel rooms. The feeling of being surrounded by fresh clean bed sheets, fluffy pillows and mint chocolate. Anyway, you don't need to rent hotel suites all the time or have a staff on hand to keep your room clean and fresh; here are some quick tips on how to perfect your room and bed to help you sleep faster.

Turn off the lights; try to sleep without any light in the room, or with a very dim light. Even small amounts of light interfere with your eyes and stimulate your brain when you sleep. Avoid any kind of noises. I am not referring to music or white noise. I mean noise from the street or anything in the room. Wear earplugs to cancel the noise and a facemask to cancel the light, whenever and wherever you can't control these things.

Something that I discovered that really helps me is to light up an incense candle. There are a few scents that help me, though others bother my sense of smell. Find one that you are comfortable with; match your emotions for the day with the scent. For example, I like to have lime basil and mandarin in the bathroom as the citrus smell gives me a sense of cleanliness, while in the bedroom I like to light up scented candles of magnolia and saffron. Buy a safe candleholder and fall asleep with the light of the candle flickering on the bedroom walls.

Turn off the TV, computers, cell phone and any other electronics. If possible, make your room a sacred sanctuary without any electronic gadgets - go old school. Have some books near you to read if you really can't fall asleep or like to read in bed. Turn on some nice and relaxing music to help you fall asleep. Or even nature sounds like water or forests sounds. You should play them on something that has a timer to turn off automatically.

Several recent studies have all come to the same conclusion that it is not good to handle electronic gadgets while in bed and right before you sleep. Not only it is dangerous because some may heat up and cause fires, some also emit radiation that can be harmful during prolonged periods of exposure. The light from their screen can also effect our eyes, while the excitement sparked on the brain is hard to slow down and makes it difficult to fall asleep.

Try to sleep as comfortable as you can. Find your best sleeping position and body posture. The best way to sleep is to keep your neck straight. Do not use a very high or low pillow while your body rests on the side or back. I personally like to add an extra pillow between my legs because it allows my hips to align with my body and helps to relax my back. Even though during the night I will kick the pillow to the side of the bed, it really helps me to fall asleep faster.

I personally like to sleep naked sometimes, especially during hot summer nights. Though some people can't fall sleep without their pajamas, some of us feel we have more freedom when we sleep naked.

Find the most comfortable way to sleep and buy comfortable nightwear that is not too tight or loose. Tight clothes can cause your body to feel trapped and prevent your blood from flowing naturally to your arms and legs. Loose sleepwear may get tangled with the bed sheets, knot itself and even make your sleeping partner uncomfortable.

Keep in mind the temperature of the room. Research suggests that the best temperature to help you fall asleep is around 65 degrees Fahrenheit, or around 18 degrees Celsius. If your room has an air conditioner or you use a heater, control its settings to keep a steady room temperature. Sleepwear is also an important factor, I usually use silk during the summer and cotton during the winter.

Buy quality bed sheets and a comfortable mattress. You spend 8 hours a day in bed or a third of your day, so why not to make a real good investment in your bed? There is a lot to choose from and a large price range. Narrow your choices considering: weight performance, additional features, price for your budget and attributes that really matter to you. A good mattress will have a good balance between firmness and bounciness. It needs to be firm to give your body a good support and they also tend to last longer. A very stiff mattress may cause damage to the skin and sore shoulders and hips, while a mattress that is not firm enough can cause back pain. Don't worry about paying out a bit more for a mattress that has an increased life span and good back support. You are worth it!

Consider the types of cloths that you purchase for sleepwear and bed sheets. Purchase materials that are more comfortable for you and to which you will not have an allergic reaction. Chose materials that do not accumulate dust easily and are easy to wash. Wash your bed sheets and pajamas frequently; it will give you such a boost of energy and confidence just by seeing a freshly prepared bed before going to sleep. And add some mint chocolates on top of the pillows, just for an extra flair of self-indulgence.

Still Awake?! Let's Count…

If all, or most of the above do not put you to sleep, you might find yourself staring at the ceiling and doubting your own investment in the mattress. Is it the new pajamas? Why is the music and the aromatherapy not working for you? Your mind might be telling you that it is time to start counting sheep, which is the cheapest and a time-proven way to help you sleep. Reality check, it has never worked for me. Counting sheep, or any other farm, desert or zoo animal! Though there are a few "counting" exercises that can really help your mind relax and zone out.

Prepare a to-do list. Have a notepad next to your bed and start scribbling down a list of things to do during the next day or week. Not only will it help you have a list of things ready in the morning, but it will also help your mind to find order and sense in the middle of random thoughts. Sometimes we are kept awake because our unconscious mind is thinking of something that you really need to do, but may have forgotten. Well, bring it all out and put it in the notepad, it will bring peace to your mind.

Count your blessings. Be thankful for what you have and do not worry about what you do not have. Sometimes it's those thoughts that keep you awake, always wondering about all the negative events in your life or all the negativity from family or friends. Turn your mind to positive thoughts. Keep pictures on your wall from a family vacation that will bring you happy thoughts or even framed awards from your work, competitive events or any other achievements.

Count from 1 to 7 as you breathe. Breathing exercises are great to help you fall asleep, coupled with meditation techniques. These will help you focus your mind and clear your thoughts. There are a lot of ways to do it, but basically, they all come down to counting upwards to 7 as you inhale slowly and then downwards back to 1 as you exhale. Keep doing it and focus your mind on a specific thought or a positive word that you like. Allow your mind to go deeper into yourself and forget about your struggles with sleep.

Get up from the bed and go outside, count the stars. I do this a lot when everything else fails. I just get out from the bed and take a walk. Look up to the sky and let my mind drift into thoughts of infinity, space walks, and aliens. Once my imagination is going, it makes it so much easier to go back into the room and start dreaming.

Conclusion

Keep a consistent bedtime routine, with a fixed schedule of when to sleep and when to wake up. Staying in bed for too long will make you feel more tired than relaxed and fresh. Even when you don't have anything else to do in the morning, just keep the same schedule as during your workdays. This will help your body to just react naturally to waking up and also to falling asleep more naturally.

Once you have found your best routine to balance your daily rhythm with your sleeping patterns, stick with them and do not let go. If your sleeping problems are too serious, consult a doctor as you may have a sleep disorder like Apnoea, narcolepsy or restless legs syndrome. Your doctor may even recommend some of the tips above. These are helpful for everyone and are healthy, even for someone who has no problem falling asleep. It can definitely increase rest and improve happiness.

Don't be lazy about falling asleep. Don't try to take shortcuts with sleeping pills and other drugs, which often have side effects and can cause additional problems. Put some effort into changing your lifestyle choices. When I used to complain about my sleepless nights, my husband would say that I actually sleep like a baby, because babies wake up every three hours! Good for him, because he actually sleeps like a rock and nothing can wake him up, even when I twist and turn in bed trying to catch some zz's.

Do not turn your life into a nightmare, trying to get yourself a dreamy night of sleep. Just don't try too hard to fall asleep. It will just increase the stress at the end of the day and will prevent you from even resting as you sleep. Remember that it's all about preparing yourself and your room to welcome you after a long day of work. It's more than worth the effort and struggles to find the perfect match between what cloths to wear, to finding a special scented candle or what painting to hang on the wall. Sweet dreams!

www.ingramcontent.com/pod-product-compliance
Lightning Source LLC
Chambersburg PA
CBHW070227260726

48658CB00006BA/2204